You Are a Work of ART!

To My Wonderful Son, Joseph Maxon Sevelitte
and in loving memory of my grandmother

PHENOMAXON

Renée Sevelitte
P. O. Box 87
Amesbury, Massachusetts 01913
reneesevelitte@alumni.neu.edu
http://homepage.mac.com/reneesevelitte/

First Edition Print

ISBN 0-9752863-0-7

Design Notes
Printed in China by Regent Publishing Services
Graphic Design by Renée Sevelitte

With special thanks to my husband, my sister and family, and the following friends
Courtney Earley, Christa Exter, Sydney Bailey-Gould
Carol-Ann McKenna, Christina Rossi, Aaron Schonberg, Allison Baginski
Matilda Halloran, Mary Kate Vasques, Kathryn Carnovale, Mary Beth Orlando
Cider Hill Farm, Cynthia Wild, Joan Klos, Joan Roberts, Yvonne Beirne, Robin Trovato
with special acknowledgment to the following children for joining in the art activities
Christopher and Samantha Orlando, Marco Carnovale, and Joseph Maxon Sevelitte

You Are a Work of ART!

Interactive Art Lessons for Children to Express Emotions

Renée Sevelitte

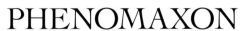

PHENOMAXON

a promise of artistic eloquence

TABLE OF CONTENTS

Introduction

Children feel different emotions everyday. Oftentimes these emotions become challenging obstacles for them. Expressing their emotions through art allows them to free up their minds from worries, to cope with their struggles, and to cherish their victories.

The text in each activity provides a gentle narrative for parents or teachers to assist children in expressing their emotions through art. In the process your children will feel calmer as they work through their emotions with you.

SECTION ONE begins with activities introducing the elements of art: line, form, color, and texture.

elements

SECTION TWO leads the way to experiment with various art techniques.

experiment

SECTION THREE focuses on expressing complex emotions through activities that involve a greater amount of time.

express

SECTION FOUR guides you to experience an art technique that can release frustration transforming negative energy into positive.

experience

Taking the first step

Talk with your children about how they feel today.

Look through this book to find the emotion that best describes how they feel.

Suggest they may write about their feelings in the diary at the front of the book.

Ask them to picture themselves as an artist and help them set up a special space as their art studio.

Help them gather art supplies and review the definitions with them.

Read the text aloud — then let them begin creating their art.

Talk with them again at the end of the activity. Ask them if their feelings have changed. Have them write about how they are now feeling in the diary at the back of the book.

Encourage them to express their emotions through art.

encourage

Assure your children their art is unique and wonderful, and more importantly that they are unique and wonderful. You may emphasize this by saying to them,

"You are a work of ART!"

Each activity suggests a famous work of art for your children to look at (or listen to) for further inspiration. This offers them a way to explore how artists through time have expressed themselves through art. You may log onto www.artcyclopedia.com to view each work of art.

explore

Looking at art will reveal to them an endless array of artistic techniques inspiring their own inventiveness.

Creating art will enhance their unique artistic style and ability to express their emotions.

enhance

—May you and the children with whom you share this book enjoy a future filled with peace and art.

Renée Sevelitte

7

Before you begin

Supplies

Crayons
White Paper

Definitions

LINE -
  a mark made by drawing

THICK -
  wide and/or
  heavily built up

THIN -
  narrow and/or
  to make less dense

VALUE -
  the measure of
  lightness or darkness
  in a color

123456789

For further inspiration look at

the painting by Franz Joseph Kline
Probst I
Museum of Fine Arts, Massachusetts

ANGRY

Thick to Thin Lines & Dark to Light Color Value

Count from One to Ten

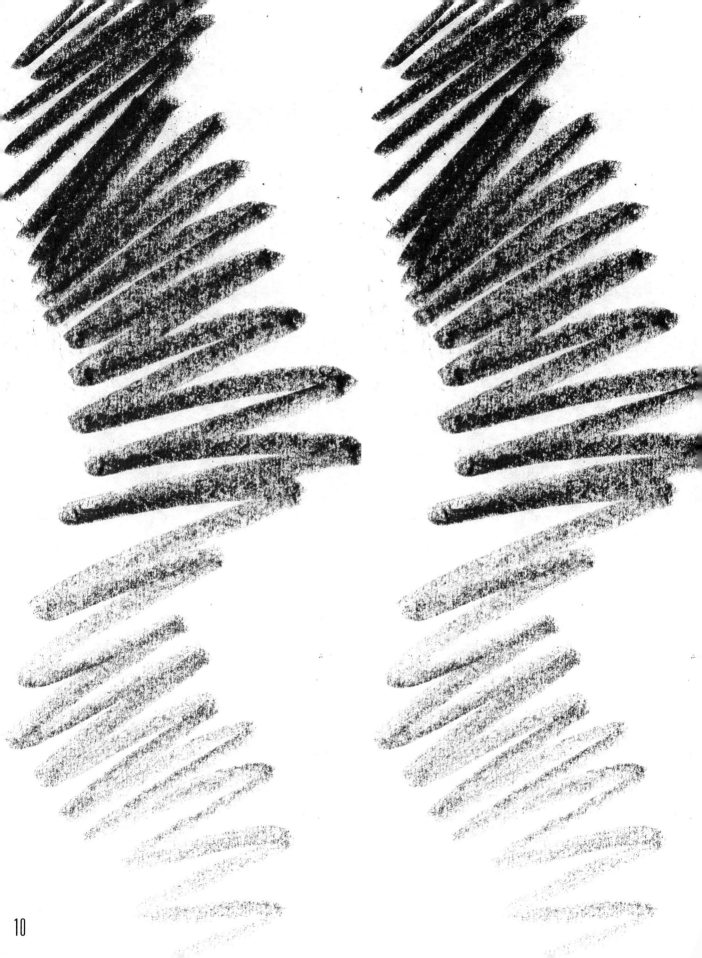

Emotion

Before you yell in anger, remember to count from one to ten.
As you're counting, let your anger go and feel calmer again.

1 2 3 4 5 6 7 8 9 10

ANGRY

Art

Start by pressing the crayon very hard on your paper.
When you press hard, the marks will appear as a **thick lines** on your paper.
Now begin to press lighter and the crayon marks will appear as **thin lines**
as well as having a lighter **value** of the color.

Repeat this over and over on your paper,
while thinking about becoming less and less angry.
Repeat until you are feeling calmer and can talk without yelling.

Before you begin

Supplies

Color Pencils
Compass
Paper

Definitions

CONCENTRIC -

> having a common center
> having a common axis

FORM -

> an area on a two-dimensional
> surface: a shape

VARY -

> to change size or measure

For further inspiration look at

the painting by Josef Albers

Homage to the Square

San Diego Museum of Art, California

HAPPY

VARIATIONS OF LARGE TO SMALL FORMS

SHARE A HAPPY THOUGHT

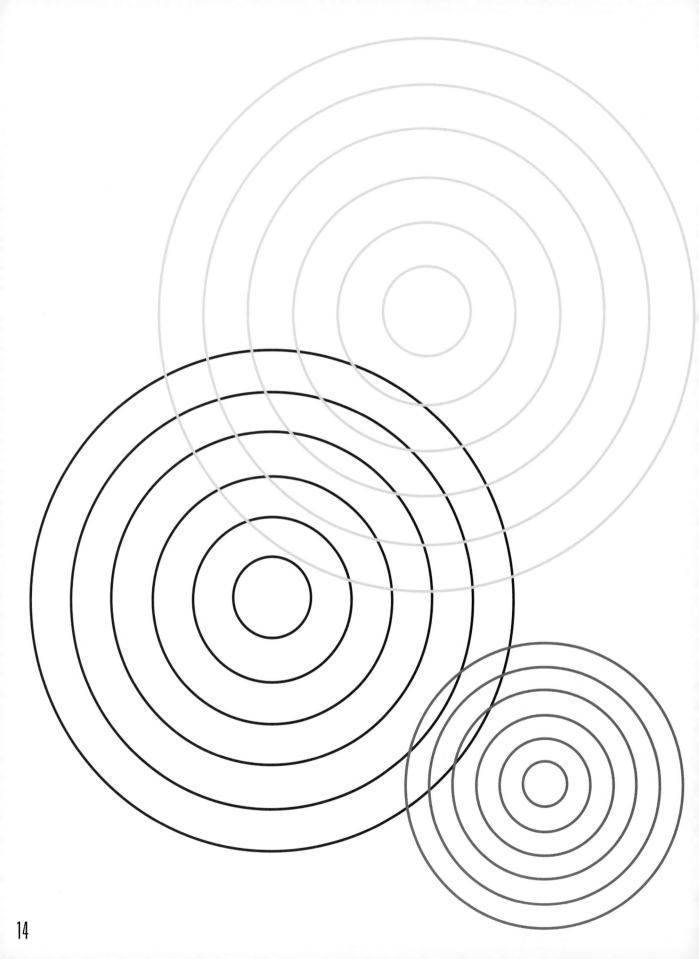

Emotion

Happiness reminds me of **concentric** circles.
Concentric circles look like the vibrations of your voice.
Your happy voice can ripple out laughter to others.
Laughing and good humor are great ways to make friends.
Sharing a happy thought may also help someone who is sad feel happy.

HAPPY

Art

Start by drawing a small circle using a compass.
Continue to surround this circle with larger circles.
Vary the size of the circle from small to large.
Repeat this over and over on your paper
while thinking about sharing happy thoughts.

A shape is often referred to in art as a **form.**

Before you begin

Supplies

Glue Stick
Pictures of Your Favorite Things
Poster Board
Scissors

Definitions

COMPLEMENTARY COLORS -
colors that appear opposite
one another on the
color wheel
(also known as the
chromatic circle)

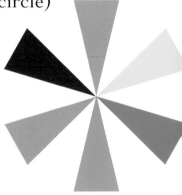

OVERLAP -
extend over and cover
one part with another part

For further inspiration look at

the painting by Vincent van Gogh

Landscape in the Snow

Guggenheim Museum, New York

Emotion

Sometimes people describe their feelings with colors.
When someone is sad they might say they are feeling "blue."
The **complementary color** of blue on the color wheel is orange.
And like the sun in the sky, orange is sunny and bright.

Let's use the idea of sunshine to turn a frown upside down,
and grow an imaginary *All-of-My-Favorite-Things Garden*.
Your garden is your place filled with things that bring you joy.

"When I'm feeling sad, I simply remember my favorite things!"

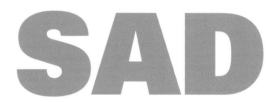

Art

Start by cutting out pictures of all your favorite things.
For instance, the pictures may be of a place, person, food, game, color,
season, activity, movie, song, anything that you can think of that makes
you smile. We used words instead of pictures — you can too.

Glue pictures and words of your favorite things onto the poster board.
You can **overlap** pictures and include small objects such as beads and
shells. Watch your garden grow as you add to it and know that your
garden is as unique and wonderful as you.

*From the song, "My Favorite Things" from the motion picture, *The Sound of Music* by Rodgers & Hammerstein.
If you would like, play this music while creating your garden.

Before you begin

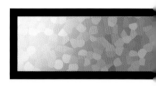

For further inspiration look at

UPSET

TEXTURE

IMAGINE A SMOOTH TIDE

Emotion

Sometimes when you are upset,
your stomach may feel like a tidal wave
swelling and rising, then spinning and crashing.

When this happens to you, imagine the tide changing,
becoming calm and smooth, gently rocking the sea back and forth.

UPSET

Art

Start by pouring sand or table salt over poster board.
With your fingers draw a tidal wave using spinning and crashing lines.
With the palm of your hand blend away the lines, imagining a calm tide
gently washing over the **texture** of the grains. As you blend away the lines,
imagine you are blending away your upset feelings.

Repeat smoothing away the sand gently back and forth
until you are feeling calm.

Before you begin

Supplies

Colored Paper

Glue Stick

Poster Board

Definitions

RANDOM -

> without a plan or pattern

EXPERIMENT -

> to try out a new process
> to discover the unknown

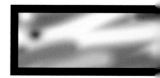

For further inspiration look at

the collage by Jan (Hans) A

Collage Arranged According to the Laws of Chanc

The Museum of Modern Art, New Yo

EXCITED

RANDOM DESIGN

CELEBRATING WITH COLOR

Emotion

When you are excited, do you feel tingling inside?
It's a great feeling to be excited about something important to you.

Being excited reminds me of confetti — because I want to celebrate.

Take a moment, and imagine yourself throwing confetti at a celebration.
The confetti floats joyfully through the air, drifting slowly before landing softly on the floor.

Your feelings of excitement can also be like confetti:
colorful and joyful *yet* smooth and easy.

EXCITED

Art

Start by tearing colored paper into confetti.
Experiment by varying the confetti in shape, color, and size.
Place your poster board on the floor.
Throw your confetti up in the air and watch it float to the floor.
You will see that the confetti creates a **random** design.
Glue each piece of confetti one at a time to the poster board,
carefully putting the pieces back in the place where they landed.

Your art can be a celebration of your moments of excitement.

Before you begin

Supplies

Cup of Water
Gatorboard®
Painter's Tape
Thin Black Marker
Wide Paint Brush
Watercolor Paints
Watercolor Paper

*Gatorboard® is a trademark
of the company Gatorboard.
Gatorboard is available
from most art supply stores.
If you cannot find Gatorboard,
you may use an alternate
waterproof surface.*

Definitions

BLEND -

to mingle two colors together
so there is no distinction
between where one ends
and the other begins;
to make a harmonious effect

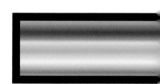

For further inspiration look at

the painting by Morris Louis
Blue Veil

Harvard University Art Museums, Fogg Art Museum, Massachusetts

APOLOGETIC

WATERCOLOR WASHES

SEE A RAINBOW AT THE END OF A STORM

Emotion

When you quarrel with someone, it may feel like there's stormy weather inside you including thunder, dark rain clouds, and even lightning!

If you've said or done something hurtful to someone — you may now feel sorry. But there is hope — and a way to let the person know that you still care about them.

First take a moment to imagine the stormy feelings inside you gently coming to an end. You may show the person you've hurt that the storm is over by giving a special gift of a rainbow.

APOLOGETIC

Art

Place a piece of watercolor paper onto your Gatorboard®. Tape along the top edge of the paper, so that half of the tape is on the paper and the other half is on the Gatorboard. While keeping your paper flat, repeat taping at the bottom, then right and left edges. Smooth water onto your watercolor paper with your paintbrush. Dip the wet paintbrush into the watercolor paint. While the paper is still damp, sweep the colors of the rainbow one by one across the paper with your paintbrush. Remember to rinse out your brush in the water after each color. Step back and watch the colors **blend** together.

Repeat this again and again, watching the endless possibilities unfold onto your paper.

After you let the watercolor paintings dry overnight, you might like to sign your name, and write a message or poem.

Before you begin

Supplies

Color Pencils

Markers

Paper

Washable Paint

*A special person
to help you*

Definitions

ARTISTIC STATEMENT -
    the message an artist
    communicates through art

UNIQUE -
    the only one of its kind

DISTRESS -
    in a situation that causes you
    pain; in need of help

SOS -
    a call for help or rescue

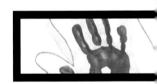

For further inspiration look at

the aquatint print by Mary Cassatt

The Bath

National Museum of Women in the Arts, Washington D.C.

DISTRESSED

Your Unique Handprint

Stamp Out Stress

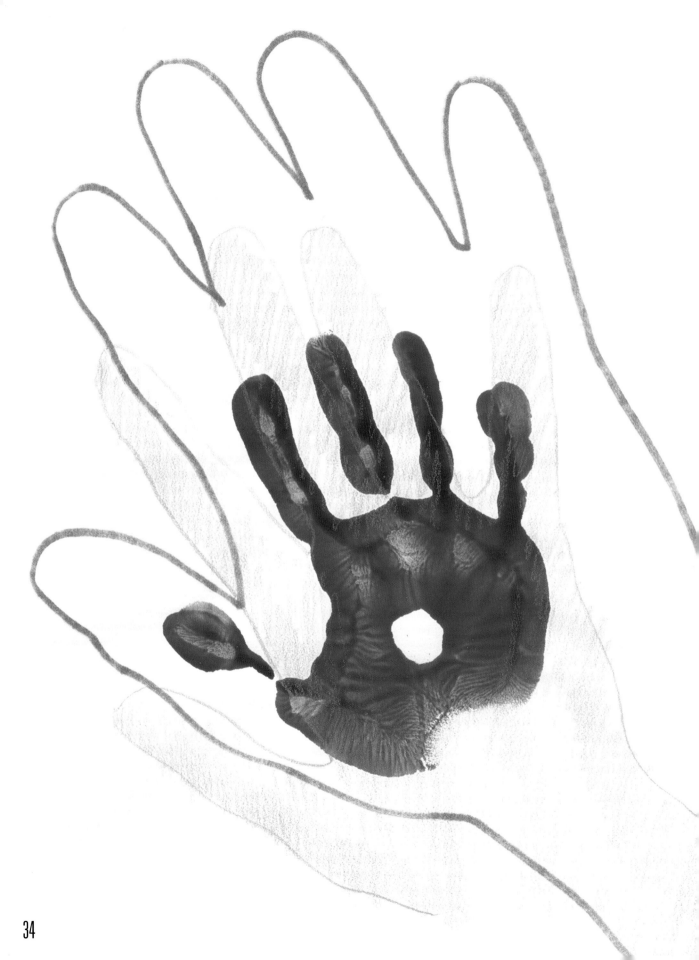

Emotion

Try to imagine what you would do if you were stranded on a deserted island.
One inventive thing to do is place rocks in an open area to spell out SOS!

When you feel that you need help from someone — that's okay.
Certain activities may overwhelm us with feelings of stress and anxiety.
These feelings may spiral out of control — until we take time to lessen the
power of these feelings and center our attention on being calm.

DISTRESSED

Art

Start by spreading your favorite color paint on a piece of paper.
Press your hand in the paint so that the paint covers the palm of your hand.
Now press your hand on another sheet of paper and say, "SOS!"
Your handprint is your **unique artistic statement** of stamping out feelings
of distress by asking for help.

After your handprint dries, bring the paper to people special to you and ask
them to trace their hand around yours with a pencil or marker. The outline
of their hand around yours is your reminder that you can ask those people
for help or a hug when you need it.

Before you begin

Supplies

Assortment of Colored Papers

Black Marker

Glue Stick

Journal Book

Scissors

Definitions

DECOUPAGE -

art made by arranging then
gluing paper cutouts

FLAT COLOR -

color without contrast

For further inspiration look at

the decoupage by Henri Matisse

Icarus

Metropolitan Museum of Art, New York

LONELY

Decoupage

Assemble a Book of Memories

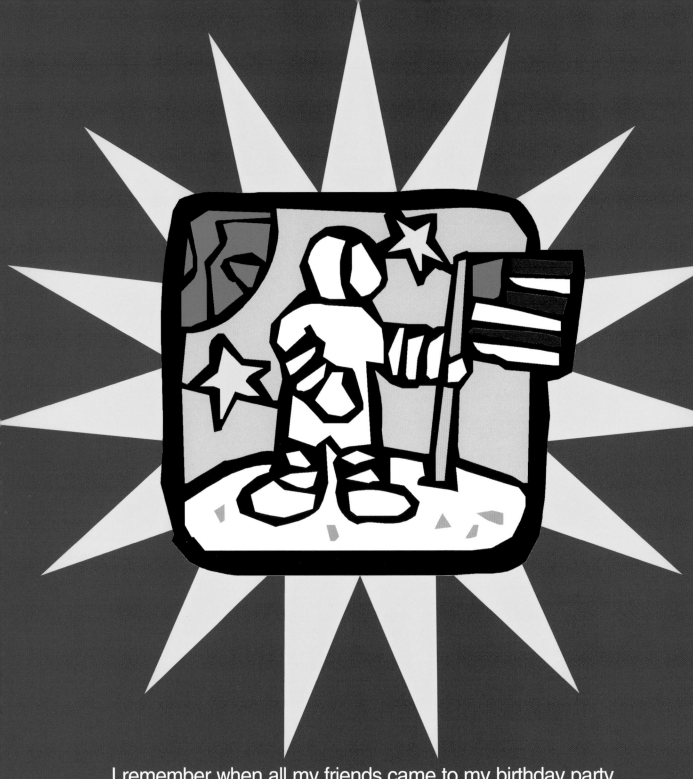

I remember when all my friends came to my birthday party.

We pretended we were astronauts and hunted for moon rocks.

The make-believe moon rocks were filled with candy!

Then we watched a silly puppet show.

Emotion

When there's a lonely feeling you want to erase,
because everyone's busy or not around,
"Memory Lane" is a wonderful place for you to travel down.

When you find that you have a little quiet time, here's an opportunity
to assemble a memory book. It can hold photos of special times that you
have shared with others. When you cannot be with someone, you can look in
your book and reflect on a special moment in time with them.

LONELY

Art

Start with a memory of a moment shared with someone special to you.
Cut out a colored paper background that will fit onto your journal page.
Cut out shapes from your collection of **flat** and bright colored papers.
Arrange the shapes on the background in a way that tells the story or
expresses how you feel about that special moment in time.
Glue the shapes down to the background paper and allow them to dry.
Glue the **decoupage** into your journal book and allow it to dry.
You may add black outlines, writing, and photographs, or place your
writing and photographs on the page next to the decoupage.

Before you begin

Supplies

Black Paper

Glue Stick

Pastels

Red or Pink Paper

Scissors

White Paper

Definitions

DEPTH -

the point of view
from front to back
or near to far

For further inspiration look at

the painting by Leonardo da Vinci

Mona Lisa

Louvre Museum, Paris

FEARFUL

Depth

Imagine Your Fear Fading Away

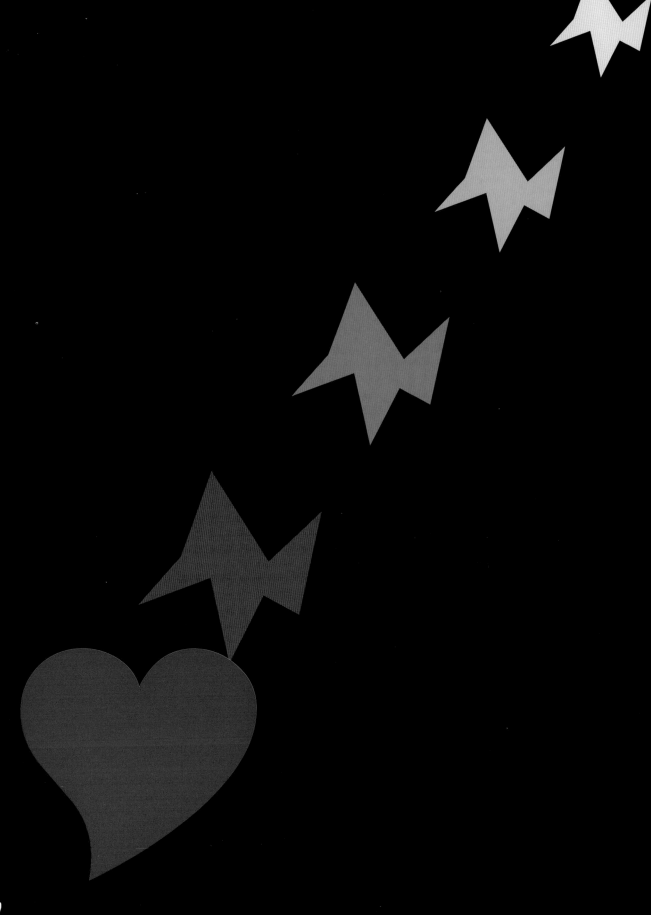

Emotion

Fearful can feel like a heavy dark shadow and can be described by different names including afraid, scared, dread, and even panic!

But worrying and fretting will not dissolve fearful feelings, only make us feel worse inside. Some helpful alternatives are:

- ♥ Talk about your fear with a kind adult.
- ♥ Imagine looking at the fear hidden in your heart.
  Then imagine letting out the fear in your heart — and sending it off to outer space.

FEARFUL

Art

Start by smoothing a pastel darkly on the first of four pieces of white paper. Smooth the pastel more lightly on each of the next three papers, each slightly lighter than the paper before. Set the four pieces of paper beside each other and you'll discover that you have created four different color values of the same color. *(Lighter color values always look farther away. Look at mountains or cityscapes and you will notice the mountains or buildings farther away appear lighter in color.)* Cut out a heart shape from a piece of red paper and glue it onto one corner of a black piece of paper. Cut out a shape from the first and darkest piece of the four papers you've colored with the pastel. Then cut out the same shape from the other papers — remember to cut out the shape smaller each time as the color value of the paper becomes lighter. Glue the darkest and biggest shape first. Then continue gluing the shapes diagonally so that they get smaller and lighter towards the opposite edge of the page. This technique allows you to add a sense of **depth** to your artwork.

While you are gluing, imagine your fear fading away like the color. Did your last piece extend off the page? If so, this may feel as though your fear will continue to go in the direction you sent it — fading away into the depths of outer space!

Before you begin

Supplies

Angle-Cut Markers

White Paper

*A sketch pad
to create unique
doodles whenever you
need to release tension*

Definitions

FLOWING -

to have a smooth continuity

RELAX -

to make less tense or rigid

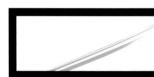

For further inspiration listen to

the music by the composer Johann Sebastian Bach

First Prelude from Well-Tempered Clavier

You may listen to this music or your choice of music for a soothing effect.

FRUSTRATED

FLOWING LINES

TRANSFORM TENSION INTO CALMNESS

Emotion

When your attempts at something important to you aren't quite working, and with every attempt you feel yourself winding up tighter and tighter — you will find this is a good time to put some space between you and your goal.

Think of it as taking time off from your struggle — to allow yourself a chance to unwind, release tension, and think more clearly. After you have had time to relax, you can begin again to work toward your goal.

FRUSTRATED

Art

Close your eyes and take time to **relax** all the parts of your body. Start from the top of your head, then move down to your neck, to your shoulders, and to every part of your body — right down to the bottom of your toes.

After you feel relaxed, open your eyes and begin to draw **flowing** lines. As your hand moves gracefully across the page, imagine yourself achieving your goal with ease.

Take your time to experience this process until you feel that you have transformed the tension you are feeling into a feeling of calmness.

You may try listening to soothing music for inspiration while creating flowing lines.

Order Form Information for the book
You Are a Work of ART!

To download a PDF file of an order form please log onto the web page:
http://homepage.mac.com/reneesevelitte/

Web Site

To receive a PDF file of an order form by e-mail please send an e-mail titled,
"Order Form" in the subject area to: reneesevelitte@alumni.neu.edu

E- Mail

To request an order form by mail please write to:
PHENOMAXON, Renée Sevelitte, P.O. Box 87, Amesbury, MA 01913

Postal Mail